The Magic

Of

COPPER

Copper is one of the oldest natural substances known to man

For centuries copper has been used in alternative medicine to relieve the pain of arthritis.

Paddy Cummins

Contents

****

"I cured my arthritis by putting two pence coins inside my shoes"

A British pensioner with crippling arthritis has discovered a simple cure for his condition – copper coins in his shoes.

The retired 85-year-old gentleman had suffered for 15 years and could barely bend his knees without excruciating pain. But after reading that copper insoles could ease the condition, he decided to put four two pence coins in each shoe to see if they helped.

Four weeks later he claimed he was cured.

"At first my arthritis came and went but then it got really bad. I saw a newspaper article about the benefit of copper insoles and it gave me the idea. I glued the coins to the insoles of my shoes and after a few weeks I could hardly believe the result.

It has given me a new lease of life. Now I am walking without any pain; it's amazing."

****

"I was driven to drink by 20 years of arthritis agony until a pair of copper insoles helped banish my pain."

A well known film star had rheumatoid arthritis for 20 years. She also suffered from the bloating side effects of medication and surgeries. She says she is now pain-free and the key to her recovery was the wearing of copper insoles in her shoes.

Although she was one of the most popular stars of the 1980s, the New York actress who is now in her sixties is the first to admit that her days as a big-screen leading lady are behind her. For many years she has had to contend with ravages of rheumatoid arthritis (RA) and the debilitating side effects of powerful medication and multiple surgeries used to treat it.

Then one day a friend recommended copper shoe insoles. She had used them and found they reduced her own shoulder pain.

"I'm a New Yorker and I used to walk a great deal. But my feet were so damaged I needed a comfortable shoe and I figured the copper insoles would at least give me a little more support. I began wearing them and after three weeks I noticed an amazing difference. I was able to walk long distances without any pain at all."

****

ARTHRITIS: My Miracle Cure.

A Devon mother-of-three feared she would never walk again when she was diagnosed with crippling arthritis.

She was so bad that she was unable to do simple tasks such as lifting her baby from his cot or getting into her bath. But thanks to a pair of copper heel insoles she was able to compete in a half marathon.

Age 39, she credits her amazing recovery to the simple copper insoles and says her improvement had left doctors astounded. She thought she would end up in a wheelchair when she was diagnosed with arthritis in every joint of her body after the birth of her third child. But within three months of wearing the insoles she began to walk freely.

"I couldn't do anything. I had to be helped off the toilet and getting in or out of the bath was difficult. It was terrifying. I was a young woman and feared I would end up in a wheelchair."

Then her mother-in-law recommended the copper insoles which had eased similar pain for her.

"I soon found I could do everything I wanted. The doctors couldn't believe I was controlling my arthritis without drugs."

****

"I lost 20 stone thanks to a pair of copper insoles"

33st man crippled by aches and pains sheds the weight in just 18 months.

A 31-year-old man has told how he managed to drop an astonishing 20 stone in 18 months – thanks to a pair of copper shoe insoles. The retail manager from West London began to pile on the pounds in his late twenties and as the weight crept up he began to experience the symptoms of arthritis. When he had reached 33 stone his life became almost unbearable.

"It was impossible to exercise, my social life was non-existent and I was often very depressed."

He was suffering from pains in his ankles, knees and lower back. He found it too exhausting to even walk a few yards and decided things had to change.

"A friend told me about those copper insoles so I bought two pair and began wearing them. As far as I'm concerned they saved my life. After just ten days I noticed a massive reduction in pain, meaning I was able to walk more. Then after three weeks I found myself walking halfway to work and halfway home – the weight began to

drop off. This was so encouraging that I started taking walks in the evenings and at weekends instead of sitting at home snacking in front of the TV. As I progressed I also changed my diet. I no longer binge on junk and have got my weight down to 13 stone. I don't ever want to go back. My life has turned around completely and I have no more pains or aches."

The apparent healing powers of copper were first pioneered by the ancient Greeks who used copper bracelets to ease pains and aches – it is claimed the insoles contain 14 times more copper than bracelets.

****

"My Copper Soles healed my arthritis pain"

Doctors cancelled an elderly patient's hip replacement operation after a pair of copper insoles in her shoes apparently cured her severe arthritis.

A 72-year-old grandmother from Somerset was told she needed a new hip due to her crippling arthritis. But the surgery was called off when she became free of pain six weeks after she started wearing copper shoe insoles.

"The pain was so bad it was affecting my life and my ability to do the things I enjoy like gardening. The doctor X-rayed my left hip and told me I had severe arthritis. I was really apprehensive when I was told I needed a replacement hip so I was given some time to consider it. When I read of the copper insoles I immediately bought a pair and started wearing them.

Within six weeks I was totally pain free. When I went back to the doctor and explained how much better I felt he was amazed. The operation was cancelled and since then I have been fine. I get the odd twinge when I climb the stairs but apart from that it has been wonderful.

Studies have claimed that copper can have both an antioxidant and pro-oxidant effect depending on the levels in the body, which enables it to ease arthritis symptoms.

****

"My copper soles healed arthritis pain"

An arthritis sufferer who feared he would never walk properly again says he has been cured – by a pair of copper insoles in his shoes.

A 69-year-old father of three from County Kerry in Ireland had so much pain in his knees that he was considering swopping his walking stick for a Zimmer frame or undergoing knee replacement surgery. But the retired printer claimed that within five weeks of wearing the copper inserts he was fit enough to play golf and take country strolls with his wife.

"The pain and swelling in my knee joints had got worse and worse. I took so many painkillers I was at my wits end. At one point I ended up bed ridden. I was extremely depressed. I really felt I didn't have a lot to live for. Then I discovered the copper insoles and I can honestly they have been a lifesaver. The healing effects of the copper cured my pain and changed my life."

****

Copper

What is it?

Copper is one of the oldest natural substances known to man. It is a chemical element (CU29) and has been in human use since 8000 BC. It was the first metal to be smelted from its ore in 5000 BC, the first to be cast into a shape in a mould in 4000 BC and the first metal to be purposefully alloyed with another metal, tin, to create bronze in 3500 BC.

Copper is a soft, malleable and ductile metal with a high thermal and electrical conductivity. A freshly exposed sheet of pure copper has a reddish-orange colour and is widely used as a conductor of heat and electricity, as a building material and as a constituent of various metal alloys such as sterling silver used in jewellery and cupronickel used to make coins.

One of the few metallic elements with a natural colour other than grey or silver, copper acquires its reddish tarnish when exposed to air. It does not react with water, but it does slowly react with atmospheric oxygen to form a layer of brown-black copper oxide.

This protects the metal from corrosion such as rust that forms on iron.

Copper is essential to all living organisms as a trace dietary mineral. In humans, it is found mainly in the liver, muscles and bones. The adult body contains between 1.4 and 2.1 mg of copper per kilogram of body weight.

This ancient metal has now been in use worldwide for 10,000 years. Its usage is increasing all the time. 95% of all copper ever mined has been extracted since 1900 and more than half was extracted in the last 25 years. The amount of copper available now is barely sufficient to allow all countries to reach developed world levels of usage.

Like aluminium, copper is 100% recyclable without any loss of quality and is the third most recycled metal after aluminium and iron. The process is easy – the scrap copper is melted in a furnace, then reduced and cast into billets and ingots. An estimated 80% of all copper ever mined is still in use today. The global per capita stock of copper now used in society is 30 - 55 kg and its importance has not diminished since it was discovered 10,000 years ago.

****

The History of Copper

In ancient times, the Egyptians used the Ankh sign to describe copper. This was also their symbol of Eternal Life. The connection was entirely appropriate as this has always been the main feature of copper and is still used for the metal today all over the world.

The name copper is the anglicized version of the Latin phrase 'aes Cyprium' because so much of the metal came from Cyprus.

In the Stone Age as men formed pastoral and agricultural communities they gradually became metal-conscious. They were already skilful users of clay, bone and wood, but those glistening particles of stone found in shallow riverbeds became a new focus of attraction. The discovery of how easily this stone could be fashioned into various shapes led to a more exhaustive search which resulted in the finding of lumps of native copper and large quantities of malachite and azurite.

The early smelting of the metal was undoubtedly a 'trial and error' and primitive practice. Almost all the ore used was handpicked to ensure that only the most worthwhile material was collected. It was then smelted down in shallow pits using charcoal as the fuel. In those days life and labour was cheap and working in the heat and sweaty atmosphere of those makeshift furnaces must have been torturous.

Egypt got its first copper from native metals and also from the large quantities of malachite found in the Red Sea hills of the Eastern Desert. At about the same time Cyprus was becoming aware of the importance of the new metal and developed its own copper mines which soon became celebrated throughout the Eastern Mediterranean.

The Romans, even before the creation of the Empire had discovered copper and had working mines in Asia Minor. They were well known for their interest in metals such as gold, silver, tin, lead and iron, and copper had become a new attraction for them.

In Britain, after the Romans had left, metal interest seemed to have waned but in the days of the Plantagenet kings the country was being supplied with copper from the Continent, particularly from Germany. It was also supplied from Mansfield and from the famous mine at Falun in Sweden, near Stockholm.

When the British resumed their own copper mining in the Tudor times they established mines in

Cumberland and later in Cornwall. But as they lacked the knowledge and expertise for the process, German miners were brought in to provide the necessary skills.

The chief centre for smelting and mining copper in Britain was established at Swansea. The Mines Royal became the headquarters of the industry, smelting and refining copper from all over the world until the mid-Victorian period.

****

American Copper

The numerous large copper mines of the United States which now produce a million tons of copper every year only began to be developed in the 1850s. Development of the Canadian mines began about 50 years later but it was in South America that the vast sources of copper were located.

Peru and Chile are extraordinarily rich in copper and it was there in the latter part of the 19th Century that mining first became a really important industry. Expansion has been continuous ever since, and with an endless supply available, new mines are being opened every year. Some of the more famous mines in this region are Chuquicamata, Cerro de Pasco, Braden and Corocoro.

Chuquicamata is the location of one of the largest opencast pits that has been in serious production since 1879 and Cerro de Pasco, at an altitude of 18,000 ft, is one of the highest mines in the world. Those mines were vital in the production of copper for home and international use. In an average year in the early part of the 20th Century the Chuquicamata mine alone produced

7 million tons of copper ore yielding 125,000 tons of copper.

The life of a copper mine is limited but in those regions, particularly in South America, the deposits are so vast that they continue to give for many decades. Some famous American mines that had long lives are Kenecott in Alaska, Calumet and Hecla, with its remarkably rich deposits of native copper on the Keweenaw Peninsula of Michigan. Since 1865 production here has been continuous. At this mine alone the yearly total of copper yielded was the largest in the United States reaching a total of 2 million tons of refined copper.

Copper mining in the United States has been a major industry since the 1840s. In 2014, production reached 1.37 million metric tonnes worth $9.7 billion, making it the fourth largest copper producer after Chile, China and Peru. As of 2014, the US had 35 million tonnes of known remaining reserves of copper, the fifth largest known reserves of copper in the world, after Chile, Australia, Peru and Mexico.

****

British Copper Mining

In the mid 18th Century, Britain produced 700,000 tons of copper. In the following 50 years the total output rose to 5 million tons. Since then production of copper in the UK has seen a steady decline.

The best years of British copper mining was in the first half of the 19th Century when mines such as Cornwall produced more than half of the world's output. To meet their rapidly growing industrial needs they also had to import large quantities from abroad notably from Russia, a country that was then well advanced in copper production, as well as from Chile.

This endless source of readily available copper from foreign mining was vital at a time when requirements were growing and when their own mines were becoming exhausted. By the end of the Century the output from the main British mine in Cornwall had diminished from a peak of 20,000 tons per annum to almost nothing.

Then in the 1930s, due to the massive growth of the electrical industry, the world's production of copper from smelters rose to a record 3 million tons annually. This expansion of world output coincided with a decline in British production. Although they had large quantities of copper ore, little was being mined, and due to the onset of globalisation and growing competition, it was cheaper to import it from other countries particularly from South America.

Virtually no copper is being extracted now from British mines.

****

Our Daily Metal

Used Worldwide Every Day

The discovery of copper 10,000 years ago has proved a gift for mankind that we have benefited from ever since. From household electrical appliances to roofing material for world famous buildings this wonderful metal and its alloys are vital requirements for our everyday needs.

The Copper Development Association is the authority of the copper industry worldwide. To promote a better understanding of copper's various applications they have categorized them into four sectors: electrical, construction, transport and other uses. They estimate that the percentage of global copper used by each sector is:

Electrical 65%

Construction 25%

Transport 7%

Other Use 3%

ELECTRICAL

Copper is the best conductor of electricity. Its corrosion resistance, ductility and malleability, makes it ideal for electrical applications. Virtually all electrical wiring worldwide are formed with copper. Transformers and motor windings are also all dependent on copper's conductivity. Most other electrical applications including computer technology, televisions, mobile phones and portable electronic devices have also become major users of copper.

ARCHITECTURE

and

CONSTRUCTION

Copper tubing is now used for water and heating systems in most developed countries of the world. This is mainly due to the ability of copper to inhibit the growth of bacterial and viral organisms in water. Other features of copper that make it ideal for tubing is its malleability and solderability. It's easy to bend and shape and it is resistant to extreme heat corrosion.

For Centuries, copper has been used as an architectural metal. It has adorned the domes and spires of many medieval churches and cathedrals, iconic buildings, skyscrapers, palaces and monuments worldwide.

Here are some of the unique examples of Copper's aesthetically beautiful application to iconic architecture throughout the world.

BELVEDERE PALACE VIENNA

One of the most famous Baroque buildings of Vienna, the Belverede Palace is host to a range of beautiful paintings, with impressive gardens and grand architecture making it extremely popular with visitors to Austria. The green copper roofs were designed to resemble tents of the Ottoman army and make the building one of the most distinctive in Austria.

BERLIN CATHEDRAL

Completed in 1905, the Berlin Cathedral is a historic piece of architecture from the German Empire. The building is the largest church in the city, hosting thousands of visitors every year from all over the world. The ornate, domed copper roof has now turned into a stunning patina colour due to the natural oxidation process of the chemical.

WALES MILLENNIUM CENTRE

The world famous Millennium Centre in Wales is a cultural hub for the arts, hosting major performances of dance, opera, musicals ballet and comedy shows. Jonathan Adams, the designer used multiple materials to create the unique structure and copper was a big feature of his design.

MINNEAPOLIS CITY HALL

Minneapolis City Hall was constructed in 1888 and to this day is used as the main government building in the city. The building was a Romanesque design with a sloping copper roof that, as it has aged, has turned into its distinctive patina green. The roof weighs 180,000 pounds and is said to be the largest roof in the country.

THE ROTUNDA.

UNIVERSITY OF VIRGINIA

The rotunda is a stunning building designed by Thomas Jefferson to represent the 'Authority of Nature and Power of Reason'. The building's structure was inspired by the Pantheon in Rome, with a large 77ft domed copper roof and pillars outside. Located on the campus of the University of Virginia, the Rotunda is used as a symbol of Jefferson's constant dedication to education and architecture.

TEMPPELIAUKIO CHURCH HELSINKI

The Temppeliaukio Church, also known as the 'Rock Church' is excavated directly into solid rock in the heart of Helsinki in Finland. Construction spanned over 30 years due to interruptions in planning during the 2nd World War, so that it was not completed until 1969. The dome and the gallery are lined in copper with exposed rock making up the walls. The church has become one of the most important and most visited architectural treasures in Finland.

MUSEUM OF FIRE. ZORY. POLAND

The Polish word, 'Zory' translates to fire, which is where the architect for the city of Zory's museum drew his inspiration. The beautiful building is constructed by three independent walls, each covered in copper plates to represent flames. To avoid the building developing a green patina like most other copper roofs the museum is covered in a high-resistance varnish to ensure it maintains its fiery appearance. It is one of Poland's iconic architectural treasures.

STATUE OF LIBERTY. NEW YORK.

The Statue of Liberty is one of the most recognisable monuments in the world. It is also the measure of the worldwide esteem in which copper is held that the architect, Bartholdi, in constructing this famous structure clothed it with the simple red metal. Millions of tourists from every corner of the world have down the years paid their respects and marvelled at the massive proportions of the Lady. Here are some of her measurements:

HEIGHT and WEIGHT

Total overall height from the base of the pedestal foundation to the tip of the torch is 305 feet 6 inches.

Height of the statue from her heel to the top of her head is 111 feet 6 inches.

Her waistline is 35 feet.

Total weight of the Statue of Liberty is 225 tons.

There are 154 steps from the pedestal to the head of the statue.

The copper covering the exterior of the statue is 3/32 of an inch (less than the thickness of two pennies) and the light green colour (called patina) is the result of the natural weathering of the copper.

CROWN and FACE

There are seven rays on her crown, one for each of the seven continents, each measuring up to 9 feet in length and weighing 150 lbs each. The face on the statue measures more than 8 foot tall.

TABLET and DATES

A tablet held in her left hand measures 23 feet 7 inches tall and 13 feet 7 inches wide inscribed with the date JULY IV MDCCLXXVI (July 4th 1776)

Official dedication ceremonies were held on Thursday 28th October 1886.

The statue arrived in New York as a gleaming copper icon, but has long since taken on copper's distinctive green patina that we see today. The statue was plated with over 80 tons of copper sheet, attached with over 1500 copper saddles and 300,000 copper rivets.

The Statue of Liberty is much more than a monument. She is a beloved friend, a living symbol of freedom to millions around the world. She is a tribute to the people who created her, built and paid for her, to the ideals she represents and to the hopes and dreams she continues to inspire.

TRANSPORT

Vital components of planes, trains, automobiles and boats are all dependent on the electrical and thermal properties of copper. In the motor industry copper radiators and oil coolers have been the standard for many decades. In recent years the growing use of electrical components in motor vehicles has increased the demand for copper from this sector.

Growing demand for electric cars will further increase global copper consumption. Those electrically powered cars contain large amounts in wiring, batteries and electric motors.

High-speed trains also use large quantities of copper as do trams and trolleys for their power units and overhead contact wires.

Airlines are big users of copper. Two per cent of an airliner's weight can be attributed to copper which includes as much as 190km of wiring.

Ship components including pipes, fittings, pumps and valves are all made of copper. Due to its excellent resistance to salt water corrosion, copper and related alloys are used to cast ship propellers that can weigh up to several tons.

OTHER USES

The myriad of other uses of copper is endless.

Household.

Copper's thermal properties make it ideal for cookware such as pots and pans, air conditioner units, heat sinks, water heaters and refrigeration.

Clocks and watches.

Watchmakers and clockmakers use copper in making pins and gears in their timepieces. Because it is non-magnetic, copper does not interfere with the operation of small mechanical devices such as tiny watches.

Coinage.

For Centuries, copper coins have found their way into millions of people's pockets and are still being used worldwide. Until 1981, the US one-cent coin was minted with 95% copper, but since that time it contains a mixture of copper and zinc as does most other coins in worldwide circulation.

So now we have seen how copper has become an important part of our everyday lives. For 10,000 years, this simple red metal has been serving us faithfully and with an endless worldwide supply still available it will go on enhancing our lives well into the far distant future.

****

Our Copper Coins

When Britain and other countries went off the Gold Standard, they were quite unintentionally initiating a Copper Standard for coins of all values. This has proved to be particularly the case throughout the British Commonwealth.

The golden sovereign was never minted from pure gold, since this would have been too soft for such a purpose. Golden money was standardized in Great Britain at 22-carat, or in other words eleven-twelfths pure; the remainder comprised either silver of copper. Before World War One, silver money was about 99 $^1/4$ per cent pure, the rest being copper. But when the value of the richer metal increased substantially between the two world wars British silver coins never contained more than 50 per cent, a figure which for manufacturing reasons was varied slightly from time to time with the balance being copper.

After 1945 the great rise in the price of silver made it necessary to call in these coins and in 1947 a cupro-nickel currency was introduced in which the percentages were 75 copper and 25 nickel.

Current 'copper' money contains 95.5 per cent copper, 3 per cent tin and 1.5 per cent zinc. These and all such figures vary slightly from time to time, depending on the market value of each metal. The three-penny piece was a mixture of brass, copper and zinc.

The total world production of copper coins absorbs thousands of tons of copper every year. The Royal Mint in London alone minted 700 million bronze and cupro-nickel coins in one recent year, representing nearly 7,000 tons of metal.

British shoppers have long viewed small copper coins as little more than a nuisance, but increasing copper prices made rummaging around the backs of sofas a little more worthwhile in recent times. Those who have 'looked after the pennies' now find that the old 1p and 2p coins are more valuable on the commodities market than on the high street with the 2p coin now worth almost 3p. But coins are not as easy to recycle and convert into new money as other forms of copper. The Royal Mint warns that it is an offence for a member of the public "to melt down a coin of the Realm."

****

Copper Craft

Adorning our lives

Copper art work is one of the most important skills developed by craftsmen. Throughout the world for many centuries coppersmiths have been creating unique art treasures from simple sheets of copper. Collections of beautiful hand carved ornaments that originated in tiny traditional workshops in isolated villages are now being displayed and enjoyed in museums across the globe.

One such village is Lahij, a municipality on the southern slopes of Greater Caucasus in Azerbaijan. The first clue to what makes this remote Caucasian village so extraordinary is the gentle tapping sound that spills from little workshops along its roughly cobbled streets.

Inside, some of the world's most accomplished coppersmiths are using small mallets to decorate plates, trays, jugs, goblets and pitchers just as their ancestors have done for centuries. They are the most visible legacy of an extraordinary artistic tradition that brought Lahij worldwide fame.

The soaring peaks that surround this village make farming impossible, so the inhabitants turned very long ago to crafts. Copper craft is their favourite and they can turn shapeless things into objects of even mystic beauty.

Crafts from this village have long been treasured by collectors throughout the Middle East and Europe. Traders discovered Lahij crafts many centuries ago and sold them for high prices at bazaars in Baghdad, Shiraz and other great Middle Eastern cities. A display of copperware made here won a gold medal at the Paris World Exposition in 1878 and today Lahij crafts are on display in museums from London and Paris to Moscow and Istanbul.

Another spot where copper art is flourishing is St. George, a city in Utah, Western United States. This is where you will find Mike Duma's workshop and showroom. His business is creating and selling copper craft to the world. His website displays photos of copper tables, cabinets, doors, water features, bar wraps, countertops, mantelpieces, lampshades, chandeliers and a myriad of other quality products crafted from a combination of smooth and textured copper.

Dumas started out in the mid 1990s building wood furniture and incorporating a little bit of copper into the pieces for accents. "The more I worked with it, the more interested I got in copper," he says. In the late 1990s, he began to make full copper pieces. "Copper just seems to be such a versatile material." Now he makes hundreds of products exclusively with copper and he is finding more use for it every day.

One of the characteristics of much of Duma's work is the combination of finishes and textures in a single piece. One chandelier, for example, is made of wood with four cylindrical pieces extending down which incorporate three different looks in each cylinder. One finish is mottled, another is golden, and another section of the cylinders was actually created with wrapped copper screen. He has also created a door that consists of squares of copper, each with a different patina or texture to create a quilted or checkerboard effect.

As he is conveniently located in the town of St. George, Mike gets most of his copper from a company which supplies the air conditioning industry. He loves the idea that recycled copper could have so many lives by the time it reaches him. "When I get a sheet of recycled copper," he says, "part of it might have been copper from ancient times."

Coppercraft Guild

A world famous name in copper craft

In recent years many people have developed a love for vintage copper. It is so smooth, rich and beautiful. When searching for quality products those who know their copper craft always look beneath the item for a trade sticker which reads: Coppercraft Guild. Taunton. Mass.

Coppercraft Guild, established in 1973, was a subsidiary of the Tandy Corporation, a famous company in the personal computer revolution in the 1980s. One of the most visionary organisations in world marketing trends, Tandy latched on to the new 'networking' idea made popular by Tupperware and which had proved so successful in the 1950s.

As Tupperware did, Coppercraft Guild loaded their reps with a suitcase full of copper home goods. These were solid copper products of the highest design and craftsmanship and were ideal for gift-giving. A Coppercraft Guild party would be hosted by the salesperson, with invited friends checking and admiring the samples and ordering them from a catalogue. Though their networking and sales parties proved popular and successful in the early years, sadly they folded up their tent in 1978 just five years after their launch.

In their short years of operation, Coppercraft Guild achieved much more than their networking and sales of merchandise. They produced an impressive array of high quality gift ware that has remained so popular with collectors over the years, and with the fashion for vintage copper products so cool now, they are getting difficult to acquire and on the wish list of all interior designers. Whatever secret formula was used in the design and coating of their products, Coppercraft Guild pieces are as bright, warm and beautiful today as they were over 40 years ago.

****

The Spirit of Ireland

Handcrafted in Copper

The Irish have long been recognised for the excellence of their handmade arts and crafts. From lace, glass, stone, marble, wood and precious metals, large collections of unique and authentic symbols of Ireland have been lovingly fashioned by creative minds and gifted hands.

For many decades, copper has been a favourite material and Irish craft people have been designing and creating amazing copper art pieces that are much sought after and cherished around the world.

Kilteel Copper Craft are Ireland's leading craftsmen in the art of handcrafted copper work. They have been in business for over 30 years and have designed and created a portfolio of classic products that have adorned homes in Ireland and around the world.

John Cassin, a master craftsman, set up the business in Dublin three decades ago before moving to the heart of Ireland in Longford where the unique pieces of copper art are now being handmade by his daughter, Michelle.

All the work is designed and made in the workshop in Longford. Each piece is individually crafted by Michelle in the old tradition using gleaming copper, polished, toned and lacquered to preserve its rich finish. Each piece carries the signature of the artist ensuring its authenticity.

Kilteel Copper Craft highlights three distinct themes in their portfolio.

<u>Symbols of Ireland</u>

<u>Traditional Irish Musicians</u>

<u>Ogham Plaques</u>

They also make custom pieces to personal specification.

Traditional Irish Symbols

Ireland is a fertile source of traditional symbols and Michelle Cassin has reproduced them to perfection. The revered Irish Harp, the historic Celtic Cross, the renowned Claddagh Ring and the mystical Irish Shamrock all look splendid in rich Irish copper.

The legendry Tara Broach and the spiritual symbol of Saint Bridget's Cross, handcrafted in perfect detail, are other examples of the artistry of Michelle and Kilkeel Copper Craft.

Traditional Irish Musicians

Ireland has a rich tradition of music and dance which in recent years has become even more popular as a result of such internationally famous shows as Riverdance and Lord of the Dance and world renowned groups like The Chieftains. Step into any good pub and you're sure to hear lively jigs and reels, foot-tapping hornpipes and lilting laments played on traditional instruments such as the fiddle, accordion and bodhraun. (Irish hand-held drum made from goatskin)

In portraying the unique characteristics of those legendry Irish musicians, Michelle has used all her artistry and the results are a fiddler, an accordionist and a bodhraun player immortalised in rich Irish copper.

Ogham Plaques

Ogham is an alphabet that appears on monumental inscriptions dating from the 4th to the 6th century AD, and in manuscripts dating from the 6th to the 9th century. It was used mainly to write primitive and old Irish and also to write Old Welsh, Pictish and Latin. It was inscribed on stone monuments throughout Ireland, England, Scotland, the Isle of Man and Wales.

Most of the Ogham Plaques created by Kilteel Copper Craft are commissioned pieces. The world famous golf club at the Old Head of Kinsale uses Michelle's craftsmanship each year to design and create special mounted copper trophies for the 'Captain's Prizes' and they are cherished by the prize-winners even more because their names are engraved on the copper in Ogham Script.

Other international companies have availed of the unique quality of Kilteel Copper Craft products, commissioning once-off pieces for gifts and presentations on special occasions. Irish copper craft is an old traditional art. With the artistry and creativity of Michelle Cassin and the expansion of Kilteel Copper Craft to an appreciative worldwide clientele, the 'Spirit of Ireland' etched in copper will continue to thrive and prosper in the years ahead.

****

The Healing Power of Copper

Why is it that so many cultures place such great importance on copper, and why is it continuing to be used today in the form of body aids? In fact, copper has been used for thousands of years as a folk remedy for many of today's ailments. It's not only a vital element for living, but it is also known for its ability to heal wounds, treat lung disorders, sterilize water, and relieve the pain of arthritis.

For many centuries, Copper has shown that it has several important properties that make it incredibly useful. It has a vital effect on bacteria as it can kill microbes. This power has puzzled scientists who can't figure out how it happens, but they are convinced that it does work. Hospital designers are also aware of copper's antimicrobial powers and to minimize bacteria transfer they make all door handles and other fittings from brass which is a blend of copper and zinc.

Copper is also a vital mineral for the survival of the human body. It has been found to regulate the thyroid, strengthen our bones, help to form new cells, and enable iron absorption.

Because of its vital role in human medicine and its amazing healing powers, the institute of 'Ayurveda', the ancient Indian health science, was so impressed with copper that they were happy to recommend its use. They believed that it was excellent for balancing the 'doshas' in the body.

They urged the use of copper vessels to purify water. This, they believed, would kill all bacteria, ensuring that it is safe to drink and its healing properties are absorbed internally.

They also favour the wearing of copper externally. Jewellery, especially bracelets, and footwear insoles made of pure copper have been found to heal many of the most common ailments of today by allowing a slower and longer lasting absorption by contact with the skin. In fact, thousands of people worldwide swear by the use of these copper aids, especially for the treatment of arthritis.

Other health benefits of copper, testified by users worldwide, include growth of the body, efficiency of iron, proper enzymatic reactions, as well as improving tissues, hair and eyes. It has also been proven to prevent premature aging and enhancing energy levels.

It has long been accepted that the health benefits of copper are important for an overall healthy existence. It enables the normal metabolic process in association with amino acids and vitamins. This cannot be produced within the body and has to be added from external food sources. In order to enjoy the health benefits it must be included in the daily diet as we use it up in our daily bodily processes.

Copper is present in many food sources such as liver, meat, seafood, beans, whole grains, soy flour, wheat bran, almonds, avocados, barley, garlic, nuts, oats, beets and lentils. It is also acquired by drinking water that flows through copper pipes and in using copper cookware.

But the big health benefits of copper relate to its anti-inflammatory actions that assist in reducing the symptoms of arthritis. The consumer market is now crowded with a myriad of copper aids such as bracelets and footwear insoles that have been proven to relieve the crippling pain associated with the condition.

****

Ayurveda

Healing with Copper

Ayurvedic medicine (Ayurveda for short) is one of the world's oldest holistic healing systems. It was developed more than 3,000 years ago in India. Based on the belief that health and wellness depends on a delicate balance between the mind, body and spirit, its main goal is to promote good health, not to fight disease.

The word Ayurveda is from the Sanskrit language and composed of two parts: 'Ayus' means life and 'Veda' means knowledge, wisdom and science. So it is more than merely a system for treating illness; it is a science of life. It offers a source of wisdom designed to help people stay healthy while realizing their full human potential. With guidelines on good daily and seasonal routines such as diet, behaviour and the best use of our senses, Ayurveda shows us that health is really the balanced union between our environment, body, mind and spirit.

In Ayurveda, copper is one of the most widely used metals. Many therapeutic treatments incorporate copper's antimicrobial properties including:

'Ushapan' – morning water therapy using a copper vessel

'Daily tongue' – scraping with copper scrapers

'Shirodhara Therapies' – using copper basins.

Vasanta Health

Vasanti Health is the world's leading promoter of 'Ayurveda Health.' They believe in fusing Eastern and Western health practices to improve the mind, body and spirit. Their community of artisans and health care practitioners are acutely aware of the global drinking water crisis and are focused on sustainable solutions.

Mantreh Atashband is the founder of Vasanti Health. She is a government and non-profit professional, experienced in managing public health programmes that provide equitable health care services to diverse communities locally and internationally.

Her strong belief in balancing Eastern and Western approaches to healthcare stem from her experience living and travelling throughout Asia and North America. Using her unique experience, she promotes holistic health care through common sense naturopathic and allopathic remedies and lifestyle alternatives. She holds a Master's degree in Public Health from the University of Waterloo.

Mantreh Atashband has written extensively on 'Ayurveda Health.' She is a strong believer in the health benefits of copper. I have pleasure in highlighting here one of her recent articles which appeared on the website of 'Vasanta Health'.

Copper

The Next 'Fountain of Youth'?

By Mantreh Atashband (August 17th 2016)

For centuries, people have been using copper products to combat the effects of aging. Legend has it that Queen Sheba was gifted copper by King Solomon and from it she created a paste which she applied to her face and body for rejuvenation. Similar legends exists invoking Queen Cleopatra and Queen Nefertiti, both known for their great beauty and vitality. Is copper the fountain of youth that we may have been ignoring?

What we do know is that the benefits of copper are endless. Ancient Yogis and Rishis have been telling us that for centuries. In 'Ayurveda,' copper is one of the most widely used metals.

Copper is an essential micronutrient, an antimicrobial and an antioxidant. It helps synthesize keratin and produce collagen, which reduces fine lines, wrinkles and blemishes, while boosting skin regeneration. Furthermore, copper aids in the production of melanin which prevents premature greying, sunburns and vitiligo. (The loss of skin colour in blotches) The beauty industry has already embraced the benefits of copper for skin rejuvenation. Look closely at many anti-aging products, even the latest shape-wear and you'll find trace amounts of copper in their ingredients and materials.

One sure way to get sufficient, safe amounts of copper in your diet is to incorporate the age-old 'Ayurvedic' practice of drinking water from a copper vessel. This daily, mindful practice will provide the body with a great boost of copper micronutrients. You can also find copper in a wide variety of foods, although normally present in small amounts. Couple those healthy fresh foods with your daily 'coppered' water and you'll surely reap the benefits from the inside out.

Some great sources of dietary copper include:

Seafood, nuts, legumes, leafy greens.

Spices like: mustard powder, chilli powder, cloves, celery seed, cumin, saffron, anise, spearmint, coriander, dill, mace, curry powder and onion powder.

Fresh and dried herbs such as: chervil, marjoram, tarragon and thyme.

Remember, the fountain of youth is never going to be a shortcut at the bottom of a makeup bag. It is a journey requiring a sensible lifestyle with proper hydration, a balanced diet, appropriate exercise and a restful mind.

****

Copper

Our Friend for Life

Copper has never enjoyed the high value status of its precious peers, gold, silver and platinum. Still, it is the most useful and used metal on earth. Nearly every major industry in the world uses copper. Its healing powers have been known and utilised for centuries and its aesthetic beauty has adorned the globe.

Copper plays a crucial role in today's society – for our health and wellbeing, as well as in our homes, our businesses and our industries. Through a sophisticated global supply chain, 25 million tonnes of the red metal is delivered annually to the world's markets. We may not always see it – as copper is often hidden behind walls or inside equipment, covered by protective insulation, or below and above the ground – but copper in daily life impacts almost every person and aspect of society, thanks to the benefits provided by copper products.

Modern living requires copper. It is an essential element for all life forms. Our health and our environment depend on the simple red metal and the world's industry would not function without it. It never wears out, is corrosion free, giving continuous antimicrobial properties, a powerful resource in our battle against health-care associated infections.

Copper is safe to use, is not harmful to people or the environment, has no added chemicals and is 100% recyclable. For 10,000 years it has been our faithful friend and after all those centuries of service we can surely offer our sincere appreciation and acknowledge 'The Magic of Copper'.

****

Also by

Paddy Cummins

At Home in Ireland

Spare Ride

Green lodge

Shades of Life

Fields of Green

The Bombing of Campile

The Crying Sea

Yoke the Pony

It's a Long Way to Malta

Dream Valley

The Long Road

Doctor Google

In Love With Malta

Yoke the Pony

Paddy Cummins

A nostalgic and emotional story set in the green isle of Ireland.

Inspired by a true story of life in Ireland three generations ago.

A tapestry of Irish childhood memories.

A beautiful memoir of innocence and simplicity.

A heart-warming novel of bygone days in Ireland.

www.amazon.com/dp/B00CPKP31E

It's a Long Way to Malta

An Irishman's 'Gem in the Med'
Paddy Cummins

The 2013 Number One Malta Travel Book.

"Paddy Cummins has created a gripping and emotional book that captivates at every turn of the page.

Endlessly fascinating, tensely absorbing, with humorous anecdotes.

This is classic travel writing – a brilliant read"

Michael K Hayes. Renowned Travel Writer. BBC Radio Presenter.

www.amazon.com/dp/B008QNJJB

The Crying Sea

Paddy Cummins

A Maltese fishing boat explodes in a raging inferno and sinks to the depths of the Mediterranean.

So begins six days and nights of unspeakable anguish for the crew; shock, horror and grief for the island of Malta.

Inspired by a true 2008 sea disaster. A harrowing story of intense human drama.

"A superb read … A story that will remain with you forever."

Damien Tiernan. Author of:'Souls Of The Sea'

This true story is now a major film

'SIMSHAR'

Green Lodge

Paddy Cummins

The equine bloodlines developed by Janet Johnson at Green Lodge Stud Farm are the secret of her brilliant success.

Her human bloodlines are a secret too, but they would lead her to turmoil, strife and dismal failure. The dream of nineteen-year-old, penniless, stable lad, Ricky Baker, to one day, own a stud farm, takes an unexpected turn with the chance discovery that his wealthy Farmer/Politician boss, is not the Sam MacArdy he thought he was.

It is the first step on a journey that would lead him to Gillian, and change their lives forever.

So begins two years of adventure, excitement, ecstasy, passion, pain and torment.

His dream and Gillian's true love are the powerful strengths that bring them through.

www.amazon.com/dp/B00B24QUWK

Time & Tide

Paddy Cummins

A Charming Collection of Short Stories and Poems.

Food for the Soul.

Stories Rich and Real.

Poems Sweet and Tender.

From Life's Ingredients.

Dream Valley

The Price of Paradise

Paddy Cummins

Jenny seemed to have everything.Fearless and talented in the saddle. Brilliantly distinguished in the boardroom. Beautiful and sensational in the bedroom. She was still unfulfilled, searching. Why?

Her handsome, older, doting husband, Dr. Ken McKevitt, knew the answer. Devastated by his failure, consumed with intense possessive love, he tried desperately to hold on to her.

Gary Wren, a stunning young racehorse trainer had just 'arrived' in the beautiful Dream Valley of South Kilkenny.

Fate played its devastating hand in locking all three together in an intriguing and turbulent saga, winning Jenny her greatest prize; her husband his peace of mind.

The reward was great, but the cost was even greater.

www.amazon.com/dp/B00G1YITBG

In Love With Malta

The Hidden Treasures

PADDY CUMMINS

Bringing you to the heart and soul of

Malta, Gozo and Comino.

Little gems that you won't find in other guide books, but define the charm and mystique of The Maltese Islands.

There is something for everyone to enjoy from living it up in modern urban resorts to wandering leisurely in little traditional hamlets and villages dotted throughout the islands where time seems to stand still and you can linger awhile and relax in the warm sunshine.

The best-selling guide on Amazon Top 100 (Malta Travel Books)

www.amazon.com/dp/B01GSFOIUI

The Long Road

Paddy Cummins

AUTOBIOGRAPHY

A MEMOIR. A JOURNEY. A LIFE.

SCHOOL-LEAVER AT AGE THIRTEEN

SHOWBAND LEADER IN THE SWINGING SIXTIES

ROYAL ASCOT RACEHORSE TRAINER

POLITICAL ACTIVIST WHO SERVED FOUR PRIME
MINISTERS

DISTINGUISHED CAREER IN BUSINESS

BEST-SELLING AUTHOR OF TWELVE BOOKS

A LIFE'S JOURNEY TO FASCINATE AND CAPTIVATE

www.amazon.co.uk

Kilteel Copper Craft

Ireland's leading craftsmen in the art of handcrafted copper work.

Founded by Master Craftsman, John Cassin, 30 years ago, Kilteel Copper Craft is now run by John's daughter, Michelle.

All the work is designed and handmade in their workshop in County Longford.

Each piece is individually made in gleaming copper in the old tradition, polished, toned and lacquered to preserve its finish and carries the signature of the artist; a guarantee of its authenticity.

Products

Symbols of Ireland.

Traditional Irish Musicians.

Ogham Plaques.

Copper Health Aids.

Special Commissions.

http://www.kilteelcoppercraft.com/

COPPER HEEL INSOLES

IRELAND

Aiding Arthritis Anguish

Handcrafted in Ireland – Relieving Pain Worldwide

The copper shoe insoles, famous around the world for the relief of arthritis pain, are now handmade in Ireland.

They are available from www.amazon.co.uk and posted to every country in Europe.

Handcrafted from pure copper, the insoles are the best and cheapest on the market.

COPPER HEEL INSOLES

(Ireland)

https://paddycummins.wordpress.com/the-magic-of-copper/

www.ingramcontent.com/pod-product-compliance
Lightning Source LLC
Chambersburg PA
CBHW050757240726
48654CB00008B/522